VEGETARIAN

DIET

MANUAL

The Complete Manual for a Fruitful and Successful Vegetarian Diet

Taylor Francis

Disclaimer

Table of Contents

<u>INTRODUCTION</u>

Accepting and making changes are never simple, and switching to a vegetarian diet is more difficult than you would think. Therefore, it is crucial to do a thorough examination before adjusting to a new lifestyle. It might be challenging to transition to a vegetarian diet sometimes. Therefore, it is preferable to be aware of both the benefits and drawbacks in advance since being a vegetarian entails much more than just avoiding meat. There are several varieties of vegetarians, some of them love to eat fish while others do not. On the other hand, some only eat fruits and vegetables and even avoid dairy items like cheese and eggs.

Choosing to eat a vegetarian diet is always a personal decision.

Before avoiding cottage cheese and other nutritious meals that provide vital nutrients,

one must also consider the nutritional supplement the body needs.

It is advisable to begin gradually and transition to a strict vegetarian diet over time. Although it may be difficult to believe, as the body won't be receiving something it is highly used to, there will be noticeable changes throughout the whole system.

Instead of abruptly eliminating meat from the diet, it is always preferable to gradually lower the amount consumed. Replace meat with fish or chicken and then progressively reduce the amount until you are completely vegetarian.

The most crucial aspect of adopting a vegetarian lifestyle is understanding the nutritional value of the foods that will be eaten in place of meat. People who disagree with a vegetarian lifestyle often think that if meat were excluded from the diet, their bodies would be deficient in important vitamins and minerals.

However, many people have been successful in making the transition to a vegetarian diet.

By giving their bodies the nutrients they need these people have been able to make up for the gap left by a vegetarian diet.

Numerous studies have shown that green vegetables like broccoli, kale, and spinach contain astronomical quantities of calcium and that eating these veggies regularly will provide the minerals needed to maintain good health.

Nuts are also widely recognized for bbeing a good source of protein. Such vegetarian diets might make sure that a person receives enough to live a healthy life with a balanced diet.

One of the most important things you can do to help your body feel healthy is to switch to a vegetarian diet. And those who have already adopted a vegan diet must have noticed how amazing they feel, how much energy they have, and how easy is to lose weight without depriving themselves. So begin to consider this and go closer to a fulfilling life.

Chapter 1

Way to Become Vegetarian.

It may seem unrealistic to consider the actions one would need to take to learn how to adopt a vegetarian diet.

But it's not as easy as just cutting off meat from one's diet, is it? The solution to the simple problem is... actually, no. People believe that being a vegan involves considerably more work than only abstaining from meat products like steak or hot.

To stay healthy and avoid depriving one's body of something that it fundamentally needs to operate entirely intentionally it was designed, and one would learn that examining the idea of being Veganism demands a lot of research and significant work. When switching to a vegan diet, the most important thing to remember to do is to go slowly.

A relaxed approach won't you've of a difference if you've been used to eating meat for years.

To become a vegan, you will need to put in some serious and thought-out effort. Start by progressively reducing the amount of meat in your daily diet.

You may go without meat for a few days before replacing it with fish or chicken. As your body gradually adapts to a change in diet, this process may gradually enable you to give up meat permanently.

To ensure that their body is getting the nutrients it needs to be well-built and efficient, a person who wants to learn how to adopt a lacto-vegetarian diet will also need to conduct a small amount of research on the nutrients that are included in various vegetables. It is important to remember that nutrients such as B and C vitamins, iron, and zinc are necessary for human health.

A proportional diet must also include foods high in calcium and protein, thus it is important to understand the nutritional content of the food you are eating. Ensuring the body receives all the vital minerals and vitamins it needs to operate properly is important.

People must make sure they get enough protein into their bodies since they are cutting meat out

of their diets. Protein is essential for the human body, thus those learning how to become vegans will want to find alternative sources of proteins so that their bodies can function as they were meant to.

Healthy Vegetarian Eating

Vegan diets are recognized to be incredibly wholesome and hearty, yet when someone follows a normal diet and is a good vegetarian, it often doesn't draw much attention. When someone cuts out animal protein and red meat from their diet, they are cutting out a major source of protein that their body needs. It follows that a vegan's diet must include items that are nutrient-dense and often found in animal products if they are to be healthy.

People may easily get the vitamins and nutrients they need from vegvegetarian sources to ensure that their vegetarian way of life is healthy and proportionate by experimenting with a diet consisting of fruits, vegetables, and whole grains.

One may get the necessary protein content they need for growth by eating foods like eggs, almonds, soy products, and legumes. It's also imporant to remember that vegans need a similar amount of other nutrients, including the vitamins D and B12, the minerals calcium and iron, and the vitamin D. However, it is true that cutting out meat and replacing it with a Da diet high in vegetables, fruits, and whole grains is healthful. However, vegetariand must also care about other important elements, such as getting the correct ratio of vitamins and minerals in their diet.

While many people regularly take vitamin supplements, many devout vegetarians avoid doing so since many of these supplements include animal products. A healthy Lacto-vegetarian diet must include foods high in vitamins B and C, iron, and niacin since these nutrients are also necessary for this way of life.

When choosing to become a vegan, one need not sacrifice their health. Consuming a nutritious vegetarian diet is not simple. One must set aside time only for leisurely research to identify foods that have the nutrients the body needs the most. You may need to read a lot of books, periodicals, or even the internet to learn about this.

When people stop eating, they may substitute meat in their diets with a variety of other foods. For instance, one may choose soymilk instead of cow's milk, which would help the body get the essential calcium. A vegetarian diet may be made nutritious by adding nuts and grains to it. Additionally, grains and nuts are rich in proteins that support the growth of strong bones.

Numerous studies have shown that vegetarians often follow a Ba's balanced eating plan results in a physically fit and healthy physique. Additionally, they are more likely to stay active and healthy. People must pay close attention to the nutrients included in the foods they consume and make sure to eat a balanced diet if they want to maintain a healthy vegan diet.

People switch to vegetaArianism for a variety of reasons, including their health, their religious beliefs, their worries about the welfare of animals the use of antibiotics and hormones in cattle, or their desire to eat in a manner that minimizes the use of excessive amounts of natural resources. Because they cannot afford to consume meat, some individuals eat mostly vegetarian food. The year-round availability of ffresh produce, the increase in vegetarian dining alternatives, and the expanding culinary impact of nations with mostly plant-based diets have all contributed to the attraction and accessibility of being a vegetarian.

In the past, studies on vegetarianism have mostly examined possible nutritional inadequacies; however, in recent years, the pendulum has swung the other way, and research is now focusing on the health advantages of a meat-free diet. Nowadays, eating a plant-based diet is acknowledged as a means to prevent many chronic diseases in addition to providing enough nutrients. The American Dietetic Association states that "appropriately planned vegetarian diets, including total vegetarian or vegan diets, are healthful, nutritionally adequate, and may provide health benefits in the pprprevention and treatment of certain diseases."

In this case, "appropriately planned" is the key phrase. Being a vegetarian won't necessarily be healthy for you unless you adhere to advice on diet, fat intake, and weight management. It's crucial to consume a variety of fruits, vegetables, and whole grains for health reasons; after all, a diet of Coke, cheese pizza, and sweets is technically "vegetarian." It's crucial to substitute healthy fats like those in nuts, olive oil, and canola oil for trans and saturated fats. Always remember you will gain weight if you consume too many calories, even from nutrient-dense, low-fat, plant-based meals. As a result, it's crucial to read food labels, use portion control, and exercise often.

Many of the health advantages of vegetarianism may be obtained without turning completely vegetarian. For instance, a Mediterranean eating pattern emphasizes plant foods with a limited intake of meat and is known to be linked to longer life and a lower risk of various chronic diseases. Even if you don't want to become a Vegetarian completely, you can change your diet to , be more vegetarian by making a few little changes, such as replacing some of your meat with fish a few times a week or using plant-based sources of protein, like beans or tofu. The choice of whether to follow a vegetarian diet is entirely up to you. Here are a few things to think about if improving your health is your objective.

different types of vegetarians

Vegetarians are those who abstain from eating any kind of meat, poultry, or seafood. However, many various types of individuals identify as vegetarians, including the following:

Vegans (complete vegetarians): Abstain from eating any animal products, including eggs, dairy, gelatin, and meat, chicken, or fish.

Lacto-ovo vegetarians: Consume dairy and egg products but no meat, poultry, or fish.

Lacto vegetarians: Consume dairy products but no meat, poultry, fish, or eggs.

Ove vegetarians: Consume eggs but no meat, poultry, fish, or dairy items.

Partial vegetarians: Refrain from eating meat but may consume fish or poultry (pesco-vegetarian, pescatarian).

Can being vegetarian help you from contracting a serious illness Maybe. Vegetarians often consume less saturated fat and cholesterol than meat eaters while consuming higher amounts of dietary fiber, potassium, magnesium, vitamin C, and phytochemicals like carotenoids and flavonoids. As a consequence, individuals are more likely to have lower blood

pressure, body mass index (BMI), total and LDL (bad) cholesterol, and blood pressure, all of which are linked to longer life expectancy and a decreased risk for numerous chronic illnesses.

However, there is currently insufficient evidence to definitively state how a vegetarian diet affects long-term health. It might be difficult to distinguish the effects of vegetarianism from other lifestyle choices that vegetarians are more likely to make, such as quitting smoking, limiting their alcohol intake, and exercising regularly. But the following is what some of the study has so far revealed: heart illness. According to some research, vegetarians are less likely to have cardiac events (such as heart attacks) or pass away from cardiac reasons. Vegetarians were, on average, 25% less likely to die of heart disease, according to one of the biggest research, which included data from five prospective studies that included more than 76,000 participants and were published some years ago. This conclusion supported prior research comparing vegetarian and non-vegetarian Seventh-day Adventists (members of this religious sect abstain from caffeine, alcohol, and tobacco use; roughly 40% are vegetarians). In another study, researchers discovered a 19% decreased risk of mortality from heart disease among vegetarians. This study included 65,000 participants in the Oxford cohort of the European Prospective Investigation into Cancer and Nutrition

(EPIC-Oxford). The observed differences might simply be the result of chance as neither group saw many fatalities.

It is ideal to pick high-fiber whole grains and legumes for heart protection since they digest slowly and have a low glycemic index, which means they assist in maintaining stable blood sugar levels. Additionally, soluble fiber lowers cholesterol levels. White rice, potatoes, and other refined carbs and starches raise blood sugar levels quickly, raising the risk of diabetes and heart attacks (all of which are risk factors for heart disease).

Also heart-protective are nuts. They have a low glycemic index and are rich in minerals, fiber, beneficial fatty acids, and antioxidants. The drawback is that nuts are high in calories; as a result, limit your daily consumption to one ounce or less of nuts. The good news is that because nuts are high in fat, and even a tiny quantity may curb hunger.

Particularly high in omega-3 fatty acids, which offers several health advantages, are walnuts.

Although fish is the greatest soursourceomega-3s, it is unclear whether omega-3s produced from plants can completely replace fish in the diet. According to one reSearch, fish, and walnuts both contain omega-3 fatty acids that reduce the risk of heart disease, but they do it in different ways. Omega-3s from fish (eicosapentaenoic acid, or EPA, and docosahexaenoic acid, or DHA) decrease triglycerides and increase HDL (good) cholesterol levels, but omega-3s from nuts (alpha-linoleic acid, or ALA) assist in lowering total cholesterol and LDL (bad) cholesterol, Cancer. Numerous studies have shown a link between consuming a healthy diet rich in fruits and vegetables and a decreased incidence of various malignancies.

Vegetarians also seem to have fewer cancer cases than non-vegetarians. However, there aren't many differences. A vegetarian diet may make it simpler to get the necessary minimum of five servings of fruits and vegetables each day, but a plant-based diet that also includes fish or chicken or that is strictly vegetarian is not always preferable. For instance, fish eaters had a reduced risk of developing certain malignancies than vegetarians, according to a pooled analysis of data from the Oxford Vegetarian Study and EPIC-Oxford.

Whether or whether you become a vegetarian, if you quit eating red meat, you'll remove a colon cancer risk factor. It is unclear whether greater risk reduction may be achieved by eliminating all animal products. In general, vegetarians have lower colonic levels of chemicals that may cause cancer, but research comparing the incidence of cancer in vegetarains and non -vegetarians have shown mixed findings.

diabetes type 2. According to research, eating mostly plants may lower your chance of developing type 2 diabetes. Even after accounting for BMI, research on Seventh-day Adventists found that vegetarians had a lower risk of acquiring diabetes than non-vegetarians. After correcting for BMI, total calorie consumption, and activity, the Harvard-based Women's Health TThe study found a similar association between consuming red meat (particularly processed meats like bacon and hot dogs) and the chance of developing diabetes.

Part 3

A vegetarian is what?

A vegetarian is someone who abstains from eating any animal products, including beef, poultry, hog, or fish, as well as eggs, dairy, gelatin, and honey. Vegetarians come in several varieties:

• **Flexitarian**: Semi-vegetarians are often referred to as flexitarians. They sometimes consume fish or meat, aalthough they mostly steer clear of them.

• **Piscatorial**: Sectarians avoid eating any chicken or other meats and only consume fish, dairy products, and eggs.

• **Lacto-ovo vegetarians:** Ovo refers to eggs and lacto refers to dairy; lacto-ovo vegetarians do not consume meat, fish, or fowl. The most popular kind of vegetarian diet is this one.

Lacto-vegetarian: Lacto-vegetarians consume dairy products but avoid eating meat, fish, poultry, or eggs.

Ovo-vegetarians consume eggs but no meat, fish, poultry, or dairy products.

• **Vegan**: Vegans abstain from consuming any animal products or components originating from animals that are included in processed meals. They don't consume any form of meat, dairy products, eggs, honey, or gelatin. certain vegans (and certain other varieties of vegetarians) decide not to wear clothing made of materials like leather, wool, or silk or use items like lotion or cosmetics that could have been subjected to animal testing.

Who decides to become a vegetarian, and why?
There are several reasons why people choose to become vegetarians. For reasons related to the environment, ethics (animal rights), or health, some individuals decide to become vegetarians. You may be able to connect to any or all of these or have entirely other motives. Being a vegetarian is a personal decision.

Vegetarian diets are healthy vegetarian diets may be beneficial and may even reduce your chances of developing cancer, cancer diabetes, and heart disease. However, when you are a vegetarian, you need to pay a little more attention to eating wholesome meals and snacks. Vegetarians often need to try to include meals that will give the same nutrients they could have previously received via animal products since they don't consume specific items in their diets. Vegetarians may get enough nutrients from non-meat sources by consuming a range of foods such as fruits, Vegetables, legumes, nuts & seeds, soy products, and whole grains. Vegetarians, particularly vegans, must be careful to receive adequate protein, iron, calcium, vitamin D, vitamin B12, and otin-3 fatty acids in their diets.

Animal nutrients: Your muscles and brain benefit from the vitamins and energy that carbs supply. Because they include the necessary amounts of carbohydrates, fiber, and several vitamins and minerals, grain products, particularly whole grains, are crucial. Vegetarians should be careful to consume a range of nutritious grains, such as quinoa, brown rice, oats, bulgur, and whole wheat bread, pasta, and tortillas.

Your body need fat to maintain wellness. Fat gives your body important fatty acids and aids in the absorption of several vitamins. Nuts, nut butters, oils, and avocados are great sources of healthful fats.

Your muscles must have protein to develop. When eliminating meat, vegetarians must be careful to consume planned meals that are high in protein. Protein can be found in nuts, seeds, nut butter (like almonds, peanut, and sunflower seed butter, soy products (like tofu, soy milk, soy yogurt, tempeh, and edamame), legumes (like beans, peas, and lentils), meat alternagives (like veggie burgers or seitan), dairy products (like milk, yogurt, and cheese), and eggs. It is crucial to consume a range of protein sources to ensure you are receiving all of the required amino acids since the majority of plant-based proteins do not naturally contain all of the essential amino acids your body requires. The only exception is soy products. They are a complete protein because they contain every important amino acid.

Minerals:

Your immune system and development depend on zinc. Whole grains (as opposed to

processed grains used to make white bread, white pasta, or white rice), fortified morning cereals, dairy products, soy foods, nuts, seeds, and legumes are all sourCES of zinc.

Beans, seeds, soybeans, tofu, fortified morning cereals, dark green leafy vegetables like spinach, and dried fruit like apricots, figs, or prunes are all sources of iron, which is crucial for the health of your blood. Iron from plants is not as effectively absorbed as iron from meat, although consuming meals high in vitamin C helps improve iron absorption. Include meals high in vitamin C, such as citrus fruits and certain vegetables, including tomatoes and bell peppers, when you consume plant-based iron sources.

To develop strong bones, calcium is necessary. Dairy items including milk, yogurt (traditional yogurt has more calcium than Greek yogurt), and cheese all include calcium. Broccoli, butternut squash, collard greens, black beans, white beans, soybeans, and tofu are other foods that contain calcium. In contrast to dairy products, plant sources of calcium Lismore is difficult for human systems to absorb and contains less calcium per serving. Soy milk, fortified oat or milk, fortified orange juice, certain cereals, and cereal bars are a few examples of foods that have calcium added to them and are referred to as "calcium-fortified." Consuming foods that have been fortified with calcium is a fantastic method to make sure you are getting adequate calcium if you decide not to consume dairy. The brands with the greatest calcium content may be identified by looking at the Nutrition Facts Label.

Vitamins:

For healthy bones and to properly absorb the calcium you consume, you need vitamin D. Vitamin D may be obtained through dietary sources including fortified orange juice, egg yolks, dairy or soy milk products, or it can be produced by the body from sunlight. It might be more difficult to get enough vitamin D from sunlight alone if you reside in an area with low sunlight, particularly in the winter. By visualizing a line connecting San Francisco and Philadelphia on a map of the United States, you may determine if you are receiving enough vitamin D from the sun. If you reside north of this line, you must get your recommended daily amount of vitamin D through food or supplements to survive the winter. You just need around 15 minutes of sun exposure to create enough vitamin D for the day if you can do so. After that, cover yourself with sunscreen.

Your nervous system and brain must have vitamin B12 to operate properly. Vegans must consume food that has been fortified with vitamin B12 since vegans can only eat vegan cuisine. Examples of B12-rich foods for vegetarians who are not vegans include cow's milk and eggs. For those who consume a vegan diet, fortified cereals, fortified soy milk, and nutritional yeast flakes are excellent sources of B12. To ensure that your body receives enough B12, your doctor or dietitian might also advise taking a supplement.

The term "essential" refers to the fact that your body cannot produce omega-3 fatty acids on its own, so you must get them from your diet. Omega-3 fatty acids assist in reducing inflammation and warding off heart disease. Walnuts, flaxseeds, chia seeds, canola oil, soybeans, or tofu are some other sources of omega-3 fatty acids that vegans

or vegetarians who avoid eggs or fatty fish like salmon must include in their diets.

A mineral called iodine supports your body's metabolism. Vegans should try to use iodized salt in recipes that call for salt since plant-based diets can sometimes be low in iodine. Iodine is also abundant in seaweed, such as the kind used to wrap sushi or other foods. Before purchasing salt, ensure that it is iodized by reading the label. Make sure to look for brands that say they are iodized if you decide to use sea salt.

Can you be a vegetarian and still be unhealthy?

It's crucial to keep in mind that, despite the potential health advantages of vegetarian diets, going vegan or vegetarian can result in nutrient deficiencies. For instance, although officially vegetarian, a diet consisting of grilled cheese, pizza, pasta, and sugar will not provide your body with all of the nutrients it requires. Similar to this, a person won't receive adequate protein if they solely consume fruits and vegetables. IToreceive all of the amazing vitamins and nutrients mentioned above, be sure to integrate fruits, vegetables, whole grains and plant-based protein sources such as beans, tofu or nuts into your diet. Be wary of meat or dairy "substitutions" since certain alternatives may not be nutritionally comparable to meat and dairy. To guarantee you are being healthy as a vegetarian, make sure you are consuming a variety of meals.

How can I tell my parents that I can still be healthy while adopting a vegetarian diet?

Your parents may be afraid that you are opting to follow a vegetarian diet without understanding how to do it in a healthy manner. If you can describe your goal to eat a healthy mix of foods and your reasons for wanting to become a vegetaIann, your parents may be more inclined to understand. You still may need to give them time to embrace your new diet. Read vegetarian cookbooks or nutritional information with your parenNTSand volunteer to assist with the buying and cooking.

Here are some suggestions for kitchen basics that will be beneficial while following a vegetarian diet:

Fruits

• Citrus fruit

• Melons

• Berries

• Fruits

• Dry fruits

dark-green veggies with leaves

1. Broccoli

• Kale

Greens, collard

The spinach

Veggies that are dark orange or yellow

A carrot

• Sugary potatoes

• Squash in winter

Legumes

• Dry or canned black, navy, pinto, and/or white beans

• Legumes

• Vegan refried or baked beans

The chickpea

• Hmm...

whole grains

• Dark rice

• Whole wheat tortillas, bread, and spaghetti

• Corn

• Oats

1. Quinoa

Soy-based goods

• Soy milk enriched with calcium

• Tofu

• Edamame, a young kind of green soybean

A: Tempeh

meat alternatives

• TVP, or texturized vegetable protein

• Seitan, a meat replacement made from gluten.

• Seeds and nuts

• Vegetarian burgers, such as those made by Morningstar®, Boca®, or Quoin®.

Dairy and eggs

• Eggs

• Milk

The yogurt

• Cheddar

What are some nutritious dishes I could make?

To learn how to include adequate protein and other nutrients in your vegetarian diet, look at our example meal options. For further inspiration, browse vegetarian cookbooks or websites. As always it is important to speak with a doctor or dietician before making any dietary changes to be sure you are getting all the nutrients you need.

*Depending on a variety of variables, including your age and degree of exercise, you could need more or less than this.

**Menu 1 uses a meal (Total® cereal) that is 100% fortified with the required amounts of zinc, iron, and vitamin B12, which are harder for teenagers to receive when they don't consume meat. It could be essential to complement consumption with a typical multivitamin on day two.

Vegetarian Sample Menu 1, italicized vegan changes

• Morning meal

o Whole Grain Total® cereal sprinkled with chopped walnuts and fruit (such as blueberries, strawberries, or bananas).

o Calcium-fortified soy milk or 1% milk.

• Snack the Hummus

o A variety of raw veggies, such as tiny carrots, bell peppers, and zucchini slices.

• Lunch

o Brown rice or a tortilla made with whole wheat Beans, black

o Guacamole or avocado

o A variety of vegetables, including shredded carrots, sprouts, mushrooms, etc., either within the wrap or sautéed and combined with the rice and beans.

o Vanilla yogurt (or yogurt made with soy or coconut milk)

o Sorbet (or angel food cake)

the Peach

• Supper

o A vegetable burger from Morningstar®

o A toasted whole wheat English muffin

o Melted part-skim mozzarella cheese (or vegan-friendly cheese like Diya® or Viol life®) on a hamburger

o Steam-seasoned broccoli with nutritional yeast supplemented with B12

• Snack

o Carrot sticks

o Nut or seed butter, such as peanut butter the Raisins Vegan alterations to the vegetarian sample menu 2 are in italics:

• Morning meal

o Toasted whole wheat

o Nut butter

the banana

o Greek yogurt (or yogurt made with soy or coconut milk)

• Snack

o Granola bars, such as Kashi® and Clif Z® bars

o Young carrots

• Lunch

o Whole-wheat bagel

o Eggs (or tofu scrambled with nutritional yeast supplemented with B12)

o Cheddar cheese (or cheese that is suitable for vegans, such as Daiya® or Violife®)

o Sliced red, yellow, orange, or green bell pepper

an Apple

o A pudding cup (or dark chocolate suitable for vegans)

• Supper

the pasta

o Tomato ketchup

Soy meatballs made with Gardein®

o Dinner roll made with whole wheat the Lce

o A variety of veggies

o Donning

o Soymilk enriched with calcium

• Snack the popcorn

o Almonds or peanuts

Chapter 2

Vegetarian Weight Loss Diet.

Because they need to lose weight yet detest the thought of starving themselves, many individuals decide to become vegetarians.

Because you are eliminating all red meat from your diet, which may iinclude a lot of fat that is stored in your body's cells and contributes to weight gain, being vegetarian can help you lose weight in a variety of other ways as well. A vegetarian consumes a lot of healthful foods including fruits, vegetables, fish, and fish, all of which may help you lose weight. You should think about switching to a vegetarian lifestyle since dieting is chalonging when you want to lose weight. Since vegetables are healthy and naturally low in calories, you won't have to worry about gaining weight while eating them.

Fruits are nutritious for you, but since the body likes to retain water, they are also quite high in water content and might cause you to weigh extra.

A solid, well-rounded vegetarian diet designed for optimum weight reduction includes a range of tasty mdeals and satiating spices. You know, the way we cook food and the ingredients we use may make it fatty.

Even if you eat a bowlful of nutritious mushrooms, cooking them in butter and heavy cream to create a soup will add calories and nullify their nutritional benefits.

As far as possible, avoid frying your meals if you're following a vegetarian diet to lose weight. If you want to sauté any of your vegetables, use extra virgin olive oil, or EVOO as Rachel Ray calls it. This oil has fewer calories and some of the healthy fats your body needs.

Additionally, you should avoid high-fat cheeses and choose lower-vegetable as well as vegetable-like likable like substituting plain yogurt for sour cream.

A vegetarian diet is a healthy way to eat and an excellent tool for losing weight. We're prepared to wager that you'll keep up your vegetarian diet once you reach your weiget reduction objectives.

Being a vegetarian is easier than many people realize. If you cultivate the majority of your veggies, you'll notice that you have greater energy, a faster metabolism (which burns fat), and lower food costs.

Therefore, choose a vegetarian diet for optimum weight reduction and watch the pounds melt off without always feeling hungry.

Chapter 3

Eating Vegetarian

Being a vegetarian is healthy. In addition to aiding in the recovery of internal metabolism, it finally results in a much better way of life.

We often encounter neighbors who need to change their diets because they have a condition that may have been brought on by an unhealthy diet. Being a vegetarian might aid someone in maintaining a careful eye on their health since those who consume meat are more likely to develop diabetes and high chgreen salad Vegetarians are often thought to consume a lot of green salad, however, this perception is partly misgreenince, from a larger viewpoint, thcategorizationon is quite different from what is typically thought.

The few mentioned categories are shown below:

• **Lacto-ovo-vegetarians** – Individuals who like eating both dairy and eggs. The vegetarian diet that is most often chosen by vegetarians.

- **Lacto-vegetarians** – People who fall into this group eat dairy products but no eggs.
- **Vegans** are those who don't eat any dairy products, eggs, or other animal products.
- **Fruitarians** are classified as vegans when they consume the fewest processed foods possible while still maintaining an optimal level of nutrition. It mostly consists of uncooked fruits, grains, and nuts. Fruitarians only consume food that can be picked without harming the plant, according to their philosophy.
- **Macrobiotic** – People who follow this diet do so for moral and intellectual reasons. With an understanding of the good and negative energy that food carries, it is taken into account. They insists positive quality, whereas the yang is its adverse quality. This eating pattern seeks to keep up a healthy diet. This diet becomes more specialized after 10 stages.

Even though vegetarians make up the majority of the population, removing all animal products and, in certain extreme circumstances, even fruits and vegetables, results in a diet that solely contains brown rice.

Everyone has different motivations for being a vegetarian. For example, some people do it because they don't want to harm animals, while others do it because they believe it to be a better lifestyle choice. Whatever the cause, vegetarians live far healthier lives than non-vegetarians, as shown by medical research.

Vegetarians have lower odds of developing diabetes, cholesterol buildup, and even certain types of cancer. The danger of consuming toxic chemicals—about which scientists have shown to cause major damage to the appropriate functioning of the body and neurological system—is eliminated when food is produced organically with little usage of pesticides.

Go ahead and take the first step toward a much healthier life if this has in any way convinced you to pursue a vegetarian lifestyle. It could be quite demanding and challenging at first, but over time, it would result in significant improvements that would make people lot safer and healthier.

A vegetarian diet excludes all animal products, including seafood. There are several variants to this, however. Some vegetarians may consume eggs and dairy products while others may forego one or both.

Another kind of vegetarianism is the vegan diet, which excludes any products derived from animals, including meat, dairy, eggs, honey, and gelatin.

The health advantages of a vegetarian diet are many. If they are well-planned, they may deliver all the vital vitamins and minerals needed for a long, healthy life.

Vegetarian children and moms who are nursing need to take extra precautions to ensure they get all the vital nutrients they need for healthy growth and development.

various vegetarian diets

Although the term "vegetarian" often refers to a "plant-based" diet, there are many distinct kinds of vegetarian diets. Several factors, such as one's health, the environment, ethics, religion, or economic circumstances, determine the kind of vegetarian diet one chooses to consume.

The primary vegetarian lifestyles include:

• Lacto-ovo-vegetarians are those who consume dairy products (such milk), eggs, and plant foods but refrain from eating any meat or shellfish.

• Lacto-vegetarians are those who consume dairy products and plant foods but refrain from eating meat, fish, and eggs.

• Ovo-vegetarians are those who consume eggs and plant foods but avoid meat, fish, and dairy products. Vegans consume exclusively plant-based cuisine and abstain from all animal products.

Two other diets that do not precisely adhere to the vegetarian lifestyle but yet emphasize cutting down on or restricting the use of animal products are:

• **Pescetarians**, who avoid eating any meat but do consume fish, dairy products, eggs, and plant-based cuisine.

• **Flexitarians**, often known as "semi-vegetarians," are persons who eat mostly plants but occasionally consume small amounts of meat and fish.

People who eat a pescetarian or flexitarian diet often do so in order to get the health advantages of a mostly vegetarian diet without completely giving up meat.

advantages of a vegetarian diet for health

Numerous health advantages, such as a decreased risk of chronic illnesses, may be obtained from a well-balanced vegetarian or vegan diet, including:

• Overweight

• Cardiovascular diseases

• hypertension, or elevated blood pressure; diabetes

• a few cancerous diseases.

Vegans and vegetarians also have fewer illnesses and fatalities from some degenerative disorders.

Getting the nutrients you need when eating vegetarian.

If you decide to follow a vegetarian or vegan diet, ensure sure it has all the necessary nutrients. This is particularly more crucial if you are expecting, want to become pregnant, are nursing, or have small children who eat vegetarianism. Meeting your nutritional needs will be simpler if you eat a variety of meals.

If a vegetarian diet is not properly planned, essential elements including protein, several minerals (particularly iron, calcium, and zinc), vitamin B12, and vitamin D might be more difficult to get.

Vegetarian sources of protein

Protein is necessary for a variety of physiological functions, including tissue growth and repair. Amino acids are the smallest building components that make up proteins. These amino acids are divided into two categories: non-essential (which the body can make) and essential (which must be received from food).

A protein is deemed "complete" if it contains all nine of the essential amino acids. The majority of plant meals, however, only contain part of the nine required amino acids, making them incomplete proteins. Among the rare exceptions to a full vegetable protein are soy products, quinoa, and amaranth seeds.

A long time ago, it was believed that vegetarians and vegans needed to eat a variety of plant foods at each meal to make sure they got their fill of complete proteins (such baked beans on toast). Recent study has shown that this is untrue.

The full complement of protein should be obtained throughout the day by consuming varied sources of amino acids.

Generally speaking, vegetarian diets may fulfill or surpass their protein needs provided energy (kilojoules or calories) consumption is adequate, while certain vegan diets may be insufficient in protein.

Several excellent plant-based sources of protein include:

• Legumes (including lentils, beans, and peas)

• Seeds and nuts

• soy products, such as tofu, tempeh, and soy beverages

• whole grains (such oats and barley) for cereal

• Fake cereals, such quinoa and amaranth

To achieve proper nutritional intakes, it is advised that vegetarians and vegans consume nuts, legumes, and whole-grain cereals on a regular basis.

Vegetarians need minerals

Make sure you acquire the recommended dosage of vital dietary minerals if you eat a vegetarian or vegan diet.

Some of these minerals, along with the recommended dietary sources for them, are:

Iron

The movement of oxygen in the blood is one of the many biological processes that iron plays a role in.

Despite the fact that vegetarian and vegan diets often include significant levels of iron from plant foods, this form of iron, known as non-haem iron, is not as readily absorbed as haem iron, which is the iron found in meat. Your body can better absorb iron if you combine non-haem iron-containing meals with those that are rich in vitamin C and food acids (such fruits and vegetables).

Suitable vegetarian iron sources include:

• iron-fortified cereal goods (such as bread and breakfast cereals).

whole grains

• Lentils

• tofu

• Leafy green veggies dried fruit.

Zinc

The body uses zinc for a variety of vital processes, including the growth of immune system cells.

zinc-rich vegetarian foods to try include:

• nuts

• tofu

• miso

• Lentils

Wheat germ:

• Foods made with entire grains.

Calcium

Calcium is essential for healthy teeth and bones. It is essential to the health and operation of muscle and nerve tissue, among other systems of the body.

Suitable vegetarian calcium sources include:

• Dairy goods

• calcium-fortified plant-based milk beverages (read the label)

• Calcium-fortified cereals and fruit juices (read the label)

• Tahini, which is sesame seed paste.

• a few tofu brands (read the label);

• veggies with leafy dark greens, particularly Asian greens

• Lentils

• a few nuts (such Brazil and almond nuts);

Iodine

To produce vital thyroid hormones involved in metabolic activities, dietary iodine is required. This covers bone and brain growth throughout pregnancy and infancy, as well as growth and energy expenditure.

Iodine-rich vegetarian foods to try include:

• bread (apart from varieties tagged "organic" or "no added salt")

• Dairy goods

• eggs

• Algae

• a few beverages made from plants that include seaweed extracts (check the label);

• salt iodized.

vegetarian sources of vitamin B12

Red blood cell synthesis requires vitamin B12, which also supports brain and nerve function. Being that vitamin B12 is exclusively present in animal sources, vegans run the danger of being deficient in it.

Vitamin B12 may be obtained vegetarian sources like:

• Dairy goods

• eggs

• a few soy drinks (see to the label);

• a few (check the label) vegetarian burgers and sausages. (Even though it's often assumed that foods like mushrooms, tempeh, miso, and sea vegetables are sources of B12, this is untrue; these foods really contain a substance that has a similar structure to B12 but doesn't function the same way as B12 in the body.)

Vegans are encouraged to take B12 supplements if they are unable to meet their B12 needs from these foods in order to prevent anemia and other symptoms of vitamin B12 insufficiency. This is crucial for nursing women since vitamin B12-deficient breastmilk might obstruct a baby's proper brain development.

The efficiency of vitamin B12 absorption declines with age, hence elderly vegetarians may also need supplements.

Before beginning any vitamin and mineral supplements, see your doctor.

vegetarian sources of vitamin D

Strong bones, muscles, and general health depend on vitamin D. Vitamin D is not a real "vitamin" even though it may also be created by the body following exposure to UV rays from sunshine, despite minor quantities of it being present in food.

Most Australians get their vitamin D mostly from sunshine. There aren't many foods that have considerable vitamin D content. The majority of individuals get relatively little vitamin D unless they consume fatty fish, eggs, liver, or foods fortified with the vitamin (like margarine). Another source of vitamin D is fortified low-fat and skim milk, however its concentration is modest.

sources of vitamin D that are vegetarian include:

• eggs

• a few margarines (see to the label)

• some cereals (read the label)

• a few milk beverages made from dairy and plants (check the label).

Since the sun is a significant source of vitamin D as well, food intake is only significant when UV radiation exposure from the sun is insufficient, such as in the case of housebound individuals or those whose clothing covers practically all of their skin.

lifelong vegan and vegetarian eating. All phases of life may benefit from a well-planned vegan or vegetarian diet. However, vegetarian diets during pregnancy and lactation, as well as infancy and youth, need specific attention. Those who eat a vegan diet should particularly be aware of this.

For extremely young kids, strict vegan diets are not advised.

pregnant vegetarians and vegans should consume

You may safely consume a vegetarian diet while pregnant as long as you eat often to acquire adequate energy. To satisfy your nutritional demands, consume a variety of meals from the five food categories every day.

Most women will need supplements for minerals (such folic acid and iodine) that are difficult to get from meals alone. Women who consume vegan diets will also need vitamin B12 supplements for their unborn children's brain development.

Eating vegetarian and vegan when nursing: If you eat a variety of meals from all five food categories each day while nursing and following a vegetarian diet, you can receive all the nutrients and energy you need. Your health care provider could suggest supplements based on your particular situation.

It may be necessary to take a vitamin or mineral supplement if you are nursing and following a vegan diet. This is especially true with vitamin B12. The brain development of a newborn may be hampered by a severe vitamin B12 deficiency in breastfeeding, which can also make the mother anemic.

It is advised that breastfeeding moms who follow a vegan diet continue to do so, preferably for two years or more.

If you're exclusively nursing or eating a vegan diet, check with a dietician to make sure your diet has the correct balance of nutrients and energy to support both your health and wellbeing and your baby's optimum growth.

Baby and small kid vegetarian and vegan diets

Babies only need breastmilk or baby formula up to the age of six months.

While breastmilk or infant formula will still comprise the majority of a baby's nourishment until they are 12 months old, most newborns are ready to be introduced to solid foods around six months.

If all of the infants' and children's nutritional and energy requirements are satisfied, it is okay to offer vegetarian and vegan diets to these age groups. This takes thoughtful preparation.

In order to guarantee that certain critical elements, such iron and vitamin B12, which are generally given by animal-based foods, are fed to some newborns, particularly those who are being introduced to vegan diet, supplements may be advised.

Children require a lot of nutrients to thrive, thus a vegetarian diet should contain:

• Protein substitutes (such as tofu, almonds, eggs, and lentils).

• Vitality for development and growth.

Iron may help avoid anemia.

• B12 vitamin.

• Calcium and vitamin D to prevent bone damage.

• Suitably sourced non-meat fats.

• Eating the right meals in the right amounts to ensure that nutrients can be digested and absorbed (for example, eating foods high in vitamin C with plant foods that are high in iron). Consult a nutritionist, physician, or mother and child health nurse before introducing your kid to a vegetarian or vegan diet to be sure they are receiving the nutrients they need for healthy growth and development.

Solid meals from all five food categories should be progressively introduced starting about six months, with the initial foods being high in iron, protein, and energy for development.

Iron is crucial for infants and children.

For newborns and early children, iron is a crucial vitamin for development. The iron reserves a baby has accumulated throughout pregnancy are often expended by the time they are six months old, therefore their first feeds must be iron-rich.

Since vegetarian sources of iron (also known as "non-haem" iron) are not always as readily absorbed by the body as animal sources of iron (also known as "harem" iron), this is crucial for infants who eat vegetarian or vegan diets.

Combining vitamin C-rich meals with foods high in iron, such as serving an orange with baked beans on toast, is a good idea. Iron is better absorbed when vitamin C is present.

These are several iron-rich non-animal sources:

• Tofu that has been simply cooked; pulses and beans (such as baked beans, lentils, chickpeas, red kidney beans, butter beans, cannellini beans, and borlotti beans);

• dark green veggies (including kale, spinach, broccoli, and green peas);

• ground seeds and nuts (such as smooth nut butters or almond powder to lower the risk of choking);

• Dried fruits (such prunes, figs, and apricots) should be served with meals rather than on their own since they may adhere to developing teeth and encourage dental decay.

• iron-fortified baby cereals

To help with digestion and to remove toxins, thoroughly cook the pulses. Young children may experience vomiting and diarrhea from undercooked pulses.

Vegetarian and vegan babies and kids have high energy requirements.

If your kid eats a lot of fiber, their small stomachs may quickly feel full before they've had a enough intake of calories or nutrients to fulfill their requirements. Additionally, the lower absorption of several minerals (such as calcium, iron, and zinc) may be brought on by high-fiber diets.

When eating a variety of foods, including lower-fibre foods (like white bread and rice) in addition to wholegrain and whole meal varieties, babies and kids on vegetarian or vegan diets can boost their absorption of nutrients and get enough energy.

Giving vegetarian children regular meals and snacks is another approach to ensure they have the energy they need.

The timing of feedings and sleeping varies from infant to baby and with age. A baby between the ages of 7-9 months' feed and sleep schedule could resemble the following table:

When you awaken, drink breastmilk or formula.

breakfast cereal for babies that has added iron

Food for grabbing (such as soft fruit)

Sleep

Lunch Savory dish (such as lentil and spinach dahl)

Food for dipping (like bits of cooked spaghetti) either breast milk or formula

Sleep

Dinner Savory dish (such as vegetable and chickpea stew)

Food for dipping (like steamed veggies) either breast milk or formula. Breastmilk or formula feeding before bed. This is only an example; your child's feeding, sleeping, and settling schedule may vary.

Try to incorporate a range of energy-giving items in your child's diet, as well as a blend of refined and unprocessed (wholegrain) cereals:

• hummus and other bean/pulse meals

• full-fat dairy (such as yoghurt, cottage cheese and custard)

• well-cooked egg

• smooth nut and seed butters (such as peanut, almond and tahini)

• avocado

• starchy foods (such as pasta, wheat, white rice, white bread and potatoes).

Use vegan spreads or vegetable oils (such extra virgin olive oil and canola oil) while cooking.

baby formula, milk, and plant-based milks

Breastmilk or infant formula is the only nourishment your baby requires up to the age of six months.

While tiny quantities of full-fat cow's milk may be used in cooking, breastmilk or baby formula should still remain the child's primary beverage until age 12 months. It's not advised to drink goat or sheep milk. Give your kid pasteurized milk instead of raw milk since the latter might make them sick.

For infants younger than 12 months, plant-based milks such as soymilk (apart from soy follow-on formula) and other nutritionally deficient plant-based milks (such as rice, oat, coconut, or almond milk) are not a viable substitute for breastmilk or baby formula.

After a year, you may start using full-fat fortified soy drinks or calcium-enriched rice and oat beverages (at least 100 mg of calcium per 100 mL) with the advice of your nurse, doctor, or nutritionist. Before introducing these milks, make sure your child's diet includes other suitable amounts of protein and vitamin B12.

To ensure a balanced diet and any necessary supplements are taken, consult a health expert before putting your kid on a vegetarian or vegan diet.

Chapter 4

Vegetarian Sports Nutrition.

Let's imagine that despite being a vegan and being quite active in sports, you are concerned about eating the correct foods.

Not to worry. You may maintain a vegetarian diet and engage in physical activity while getting all the nourishment you need. Just because you don't want to eat meat doesn't mean you have to change your diet.

In fact, you could discover that a vegetarian diet makes it quite easy for you to engage in physical activity since the nutrients in grains, vegetables, and other plant foods really offer you greater energy. The first thing you should keep in mind is that you must eat before exercising so that your body can start processing the food and provide you with the nourishment you need to survive a rigorous exercise and have the energy to engage in the sports you like.

This implies that vegetarians must consume a lot of carbs before to engaging in physical activity so that the nutrients included in those meals can do its job.

In order to replace the nutrients that is naturally lost via perspiration during your exercise, you should have a healthy vegetarian meal right after you finish engaging in your sport.

However, you should try to limit the amount of carbohydrates you eat during this meal since they may quickly turn into fat, negating all the advantages you have just given yourself.

If you are a lacto-vegetarian who is actively involved in sports, we advise you to consume a lot of nuts, grains, and fruits. These foods are rich in carbohydrates and can help your body replenish the water it will eventually lose through sweat.

Since exercise is so crucial to staying in shape, vegetarian athletes often worry about their diet. All they actually need to keep in mind is that certain vitamins and minerals are necessary for the body to operate properly. When it comes to it, research is important.

In order to prevent their nutrition from suffering, ask some of your vegetarian friends what they do before to participating in sports. Look online for tips on how to maximize the nutrients in your vegetarian diet before engaging in physical activity.

If you're a vegetarian who does a lot of sports and you're concerned about nutrition, read books and see your doctor along the way. You can never have too much knowledge, so look for what's available to you and then pay attention. In the end, it will all be worthwhile!

It is possible for an athlete to follow a vegan or vegetarian diet without suffering from performance or body composition issues, but doing so requires preparation and deliberate food selection. This article may assist plant-based athletes manage meal planning for performance by acting as a nutrition guide.

Become a sports nutrition coach now to provide qualified nutritional guidance that is tailored to sports nutrition!

VEGETARIAN ATHLETES' NUTRITIONAL NEEDS

A plant-based diet known as a vegan diet forgoes the intake of any animal products, such as meat, fish, eggs, and dairy. For the nutrients that these foods supply, including as plant-based protein sources and crucial micronutrients like vitamin B12 and calcium, the vegan athlete must find substitute sources.

NEEDS FOR MICRONUTRIENTS

Vitamins and minerals that the body needs in extremely tiny quantities are known as micronutrients. Generally speaking, a variety of meals may be eaten to provide these essential elements. Finding substitute sources to satisfy the body's micronutrient requirements is important when following a diet that forbids the consumption of specific foods, such as a vegan one.

B12 VITAMIN

The creation of DNA, cell metabolism, brain function, and red blood cell development are all aided by vitamin B12 .

B12 supplements are the best source for vegans.

OMEGAFATTY ACIDS, GLA-3 Omega-3 fatty acids are critical for heart health, lowering blood pressure and heart rate, improving blood vessel function, and reducing inflammation.

The best vegan source is EPA/DHA supplements, which are sold over-the-counter and derived from microalgae.

CALCIUM

Calcium is essential for more than simply having strong, healthy bones, according to the National Osteoporosis. Our muscles can contract, our blood can clot, and our heart can beat thanks to it.

Leafy green veggies are the best vegan supply.

IRON

Iron aids in delivering oxygen to the body's tissues so they may be used for metabolism.

Dark leafy greens, lentils, and dried fruit are the best vegan sources. It's vital to keep in mind that these iron sources are not as easily absorbed by the body as animal sources. Include foods high in vitamin C in your diet to enhance absorption, such as oranges, pineapples, red and green bell peppers, kale, Brussels sprouts, and cabbage (Lynch & Cook, 1980).

NEEDS FOR MACRONUTRIENTS

The macronutrients, or nutrients that your body utilizes in the greatest quantities, are protein, fat, and carbs. To support our health and athletic objectives, we must consume these nutrients in the right amounts from the foods we eat.

PROTEIN

Protein is crucial for more than just muscle growth and repair; it also gives the body's other tissues, including cell membranes, organs, blood plasma, hair, skin, and nails, as well as its bones, tendons, ligaments, and skin.

Protein intake goals of 0.7 to 1.0 grams per pound are suitable for athletes or those who want to optimize muscle development and training responses. Lentils, beans, soy products, nuts, seeds, and whole grains are vegan sources of protein.

We need fat to absorb fat-soluble vitamins, act as a reservoir of energy, and protect and insulate our organs. Healthy fats such as vegetable oils (olive, canola, and avocado oil), avocado, flax seeds, chia seeds, olives, nuts, and seeds should make up 20–35% of your daily calorie intake. Because athletes need more carbohydrates, their fat consumption will often be on the lower end of the range.

CARBOHYDRATES

All people need carbohydrates as their primary source of energy, and athletes depend heavily on them. Depending on how hard and how long they exercise, athletes may get between 40 and 65 percent of their energy from carbs.

You will need to eat more carbs the more often and intensely you exercise.

SPECIFIC VEGAN FOOD SOURCES TO BUILD MUSCLE

Vegan athletes must make sure they are consuming enough calories throughout the day and getting enough protein to develop muscle. To do this, it may be essential to consume many meals (3-5) during the day. Examples of plant-based protein sources include:

20g of tofu per cup.

15g of tempeh per half cup

Beans/lentils: 7-8g per serving of 12 cup

Hemp seeds: 1 ounce contains 9.5g.

squash seeds 8.5 grams per ounce

8g of nut butter per 2 TBSP

Grains: for cooked 12 cup, 3-5 grams

In order to boost their protein intake for growing muscle, athletes may also think about consuming a portion of vegan protein powder once a day.

VEGETARIAN Athletes' NUTRITIONAL NEEDSAn athlete who practices vegetarianism avoids eating meat, fish, and fowl. Vegetarianism comes in a variety of forms, including:

Vegetarian who consumes dairy and eggs but avoids meat, fish, and poultry.

A lacto-vegetarian permits dairy products but forgoes meat, fish, poultry, and eggs. Ovo-vegetarians include eggs but forego meat, fish, poultry, and dairy items.

Pescatarians forgo meat and poultry in favor of fish, sometimes eggs, and dairy products.

NEEDS FOR MICRONUTRIENTS

Vegetarian diets may also be lacking in vitamin B12, DHA/EPA, calcium, and iron, just as vegan diets can. Vegetarians may get enough calcium from dairy products or leafy greens; however, vegetarians will need to take supplements for vitamin B12 and DHA/EPA. EPA/DHA may be found in fatty fish like salmon, mackerel, sea bass, or sardines, which are options for sectarians. Athletes who are vegetarians require the same quantities of macronutrients as vegan athletes, but they have more protein alternatives since they can eat fish, dairy products, eggs, and other lean meats.

SAMPLE DIET PLAN FOR ATHLETES
BASED ON PLANT FOODS

Use the plate-construction strategy to make dinner preparation easier.

Take your protein first. Put a plant-based protein on one-third of your dish.

Black beans, kidney beans, tofu, or lentils are suitable for vegans.

Eggs, Greek yogurt, cottage cheese, or fish may all be options for vegetarians.

Add carbs next. Your plate will have a plant-based carbohydrate (such as whole

grains, starchy vegetables, and/or fruit) in the proportion of around one-quarter to one-third. You may add fewer food sources in this area of your plate if your protein source has a higher carb content (such as beans and lentils).

Vegetables without starch come next. Non-starchy veggies like leafy greens, bell peppers, zucchini, broccoli, cauliflower, etc. should take up the remaining space on your plate.

Add a serving of a good fat last. 1 teaspoon oil, 14 an avocado, and a tiny handful of nuts or seeds.

You may have your meal as specified on a plate, or for variation, try mixing the items in a bowl, producing soups, smoothies, or salads. You will be able to consume a range of prepared and uncooked sources of plant-based meals thanks to these many meal alternatives!

IS A PLANT-BASED DIET MORE EFFECTIVE AND WHY AREN'T ALL ATHLETES VEGANS?

An athlete makes nutrition decisions depending on their dietary preferences, practicality, and sustainability. Eliminating foods made from animals doesn't seem viable to some people. Others prefer consuming animal-based foods over their vegan or vegetarian counterparts because of their flavor and convenience.

Although plant-based diets are excellent for losing weight and have many positive effects on your health and way of life, they may not meet your specific demands as an athlete.

THE BENEFITS AND POSSIBLE CONS OF BEING A PLANT-BASED ATHLETE

Pros:

When a vegan or vegetarian diet primarily consists of plant-based foods and little processed food, it may have numerous positive health effects. It is undeniably true that diets heavy in fruits and vegetables are healthier than those high in processed meat and other processed foods. The tendency of vegan and vegetarian diets to have more carbs is also advantageous for performance.

Cons:

In order to maximize performance and health, vegan or vegetarian athletes will need to pay more attention to consuming enough protein and calories. As a vegan or vegetarian, it's simpler to go short on crucial minerals, protein, and calories, all of which may affect health and performance. Due to the restricted dietary alternatives available while traveling regularly for competition, it could be more difficult to maintain a plant-based diet.

Chapter 5

Vegetarian Cooking for Everyone

It is true that cooking vegetarian meals is among the simplest skills to acquire. Vegetarian cuisine is incredibly intriguing and simple to make, even for people who are afraid of boiling water or preparing food. Everyone can prepare vegetarian food. In addition to being very nutritious, vegetarian cooking is simple for everyone.

The best-selling book "Vegetarian Cooking for Everyone" was just released by America's top chef, Deborah Madison. You shouldn't consider it to be another cookbook for vegetarians. It includes 800 scrumptious recipes as well as crucial information on the elements and techniques of cooking.

The book teaches innovative techniques for making well-known foods like guacamole as well as obscure ones like green lentils with roasted beets and preserved lemons and cashew curry.

The 124-page chapter on veggies, titled "The Heart of Matter," may be used as a reference for any vegetarian culinary abilities, according to one Amazon review. It may have been used as a guide or as assistance while purchasing veggies. "Madison provides equally inspired recipes and guidance for everything from grains and soy to dairy foods and desserts." It has proven to be an excellent resource and has made learning enjoyable for all of its readers. One reviewer even admitted that the author's writing on recipes for the typical kitchen is what draws readers of all ages. It's not like those chef books where the reader or student finds it challenging to cook the recipes.

Everyone should read "Vegetarian Cooking for Everyone." Even a mediocre chef who reads from it may plan or cook delicious meals. A novice or new learner who can successfully create tasty vegetarian meals will find this to be of great assistance as it will boost his confidence. It has been determined that "Vegetarian Cooking for Everyone" is a thorough book that is interesting to everyone, including those who wish to use it as a resource for regular cooking. Every meal is covered, including appetizers, sizzlers, snacks, breakfast, lunch, and supper.

It's easy to find the ingredients in one's cupboard and refrigerator, and using them to make something delicious is quite satisfying and enjoyable.

This book teaches everyone the fundamentals of vegetarian cookery. So read the book and have fun!

Gourmet Vegetarian Cooking

There are a ton of chances for vegans who like preparing upscale foods to explore and discover. You can prepare a large variety of epicurean vegan foods in a variety of settings and circumstances; you simply need to look for opportunities.

Unfortunately, due to space restrictions, we are unable to include every cookbook available in this brief post. However, there are a few suggestions I can provide for great vegetarian meal preparation.

First, let's define an epicurean meal. Now, the issue of feasibility emerges. A gourmet lunch is really a special meal without meat or pasta that involves combining unusual and uncommon ingredients to create meals that are not only tasty but also visually stunning.

Gourmet may be defined in a variety of ways, but making gourmet vegan cuisine requires a certain level of skill. It demands a lot of taste and the capacity to transform ordinary components into works of beauty.

So what information is required to prepare a gourmet vegetarian meal? If they have been a lacto-vegetarian for a while, they may want to think about what they like eating and how to add creativity to make it interesting and delectable in addition to scrumptious.

The greatest method for introducing vegetarian food to individuals is to think about the kinds of gourmet meals they have previously enjoyed. It is absolutely true that practically all of us have eaten vegetarian meals. It's important to always explore for methods to make a meal without the meat and keep the flavor intact.

We know virtually everyone can do this with a little creativity and ingenuity!

In their local bookshop, online, on other websites, and elsewhere, one may locate sizable and varied recipe books that are wholly devoted to gourmet vegetarian cuisine. Search for culinary techniques that use ingredients that everyone find fascinating before trying the dish.

If they begin from anywhere, many people will not be able to prepare a gourmet vegetarian feast. However, if you strictly adhere to the directions, you may avoid a culinary disaster.

Being a vegan chef, preparing a gourmet dinner may be a very exciting and revitalizing experience. Many people think that living a vegetarian lifestyle requires confusion and curiosity. When one can simply show that they are capable of providing a vegetarian meal that is exquisite, visually appealing, and delicious, they may just wave them over to their side of the fence.

But don't push yourself too far. A lacto-vegetarian lifestyle is not for everyone. The best thing someone can do is cook from the heart and stick to their commitment to leading a vegetarian lifestyle, which involves creating gourmet dishes that taste like they include mutton but don't really contain any meat.

Chapter 6

Vegetarian Low Carb

The body needs a variety of nutrients to be healthy. Being a vegetarian is beneficial, but you must carefully balance the vitamins and minerals.

The carbohydrate balance should be the sole thought that enters your head. Only because carbohydrates are such a tremendous source of energy should they be used in moderation. An excessive amount of carbohydrates in a vegetarian diet will cause the body to produce fat. Carbs transform sugar, which then turns into fat, which might be problematic if there is an excessive amount of conversion.

If you want to reduce your intake of carbs, you should limit your intake of foods high in carbohydrates such rice, potatoes, and cereals. Since these foods are an excellent source of carbohydrates, it is also not suggested to fully exclude them from your diet. The intake of certain food items has to be reduced.

Additionally, flour contains carbs, even whole wheat flour. If you are serious about getting the right amount of carbohydrates, you should avoid or limit eating bread. To regulate the right intake of carbohydrates, ensure that the source of your carbohydrates is acceptable. Eat whole grain bread instead of white bread to satisfy your body's need for carbohydrates. Being a vegetarian is beneficial, but it requires a lot of sacrifices.

There should be a large amount of fresh, green vegetables in the diet.

Additionally, consideration should be given to the choice of oils used in food preparation. To get the necessary amount of carbs, you must use the right amount of olive oil. To guarantee a reduced carb consumption, also take into account steaming and grilling with oil. Green and leafy veggies provide natural vitamins. Avoid consuming carbs that may cause you to gain weight.

The decision to choose a vegetarian diet varies among individuals for a variety of reasons. The primary motivation is shedding additional weight. Others are really worried about the slaughter of numerous animals. The main need for leading a vegetarian lifestyle is a healthy diet. An excessive intake of carbs may convert to sugar, which can progressively result in weight gain.

You must be extremely cautious to determine the precise quantity of carbohydrates available in your diet before beginning a vegetarian diet that is similarly low in carbohydrate content. Low carbohydrate intake may have an impact on your body, and most crucially, your health. Nutrition is the most crucial component of a healthy diet.

Recipes for Low-Calorie Vegetarian Food.

Perhaps someone who wanted to lose weight would have chosen a vegetarian way of life and needed a vegan diet low in calories to help them achieve their goals. The great news is that reducing one's intake of meat would result in reduced calorie consumption. The secret to making healthy vegan dishes is getting rid of the extra fat that makes meals substantial.

When making low-fat vegan dishes, folks should first try to avoid using a lot of oil. For salads and tastings, one may still use extra virgin olive oil of the highest quality. EVOO provides some of the "beneficial fats" that our bodies need while having a lower calorie value.

While preparing vegetarian dishes with lower calorie counts, avoid eating fried items. Even if one does use the extra virgin olive oil for frying, one should avoid fried dishes as much as is practical since they often contain more calories.

Steer clear of boiling the veggies and instead steam them. Significant nutrients will be lost while boiling. For a change, grill some veggies. To give them some moisture, you may also spritz on a low-calorie or light cooking spray, or even sprinkle some watery lemon juice on top.

If one must consume seafood due to their diet, boil the fish rather than frying it. It is recommended to grill the fish since it is a great way to add flavor and uniqueness to cuisine. Spices are key components that may make a significant difference and provide a delicious and enticing low-fat vegetarian dish.

Online resources abound for low-calorie vegetarian cooking. Cookbooks for vegetarians that include low-fat recipes are also available. Simple substitutions like diet cheeses or plain yogurt for vinegary cream are a more efficient and practical way to create vegetarian dishes that are low in calories.

If a person is inventive, they will be astounded to learn that there are a ton of nutritious vegetarian meals available, and that they may include these recipes into their diets to balance their weight reduction goals.

All it takes is a little knowledge about substitutions that may be made to change high-calorie dishes into low-calorie foods with a little variety and plenty of thinking. Adopt low-calorie vegan dishes into your regular diet and realize that you may enjoy delectable cuisine while maintaining your vegetarian lifestyle.

Chapter 7

Vegetarian Vegan

Since the dietary habits of vegetarians and non-vegetarians are unique and evident, the distinction between the two is well known.

The distinction between vegetarianism and veganism is erroneously made, and there is another branch of the food-eating community that is often known as vegan. Although there are no obvious differences between vegan and vegetarian eating styles, many still struggle to classify these dietary eating groups.

You won't be able to distinguish between vegetarian and vegan diets as a layperson. Because of their evident and obvious connections, many see them as belonging to the same food consumption groups.

People like to believe what they see, therefore it's common to observe a vegetarian consuming fresh green salads and a few broccoli for each of their three meals. In actuality, not all vegetarians and vegans eat food in the same manner and their practices are not necessarily complementary. Things will become evident after you are aware of this faction's feeding habits. Here are a few instances:

Lacto-ovo-vegetarians are people who eat dairy products, eggs, fruits, and vegetables. One of the most popular and common types of lacto-vegetarian diet is this one. These groups sometimes consume both fish and goods made from chicken.

Lacto-vegetarians use dairy products, cereals, fruits, vegetables, and healthy nuts in their diet. The sole distinction is that this group doesn't eat eggs.

Vegans: By observing their eating patterns, we can distinguish between vegans and vegetarians. Vegans refrain from consuming dairy products, eggs, or any other kind of animal products in their daily diet.

These vegans have abstained from wearing or sporting anything made from animal products.

Follow a diet group for a variety of reasons, including macrobiotics. Macrobiotic diet refers to a way of eating based on philosophy and spirituality. Before choosing this diet, health-related considerations are also taken into consideration. Foods

are divided into negative and positive categories in this diet. Yang is the negative group, whereas eying is the good group. This diet has many progression stages. At all levels, the use of animal products is promoted. The strictest level restricts consumption to just brown rice and bans even fruits and vegetables. A typical individual would undoubtedly mix up the vegetarian and lacto-vegetarian diets. However, adopting a vegan or vegetarian lifestyle is really simple. The benefits and drawbacks of a diet regimen become clear only once you begin to adhere to it. As long as it's healthy and keeps you strong, you need to embrace all dietary ideologies and eating practices. What exactly are vegan and vegetarian diets?

Diets that are vegetarian and vegan can lower your risk of illness. Additionally, they may provide you all the protein, minerals, and the majority of the vitamins your body requires.

Vegans avoid eating any meat, poultry, or seafood. There are several kinds of vegetarian diets, though: Lacto-ovo vegetarians consume dairy and eggs.

• Vegans abstain from consuming any animal products, such as honey and gelatin.

Sectarians concentrate on a diet rich in plants but are not entirely vegetarians since they consume fish. People may choose a vegetarian or vegan diet because of ethical or ecological considerations or for religious reasons. What advantages does a vegetarian diet provide for your health?

When properly planned, vegetarian diets may also be beneficial to your health. Vegetarian diets rich in fruits, vegetables, whole grains, legumes, beans, nuts, and seeds may help lower the risk of:

• Heart conditions

Blood pressure problems

• Diabetes type 2

• Overweight

• a few forms of cancer; gallstones

• gout

• Kidney illness

Diverticular illness

The 'healthy' bacteria in your gut are increased by dietary fiber in a plant-based diet. That may:

• enhance intestinal wellness

• minimize irritation

How can I eat a vegetarian diet and yet satisfy my nutritional needs?

Your nutritional demands may be satisfied by a well-planned vegetarian diet that consists of a wide range of plant-based foods. Foods from the five food categories are included in this.

Some nutrients, meanwhile, could need extra care.

Particularly in the case of children's meals, a vegan diet need additional attention to guarantee that your body receives sufficient nutrients.

Here's how you eat a vegetarian or vegan diet and still get enough protein, calcium, iron, and other minerals.

Protein

Amino acids make up protein. In the body, essential amino acids cannot be produced. Meat, poultry, fish, eggs, milk, cheese, and yoghurt are some common sources of them.

The necessary amino acids are not all present in every plant. However, by consuming a variety of plant-based protein

sources every day, you may get all the amino acids you need.

Among the best sources of protein are:

• Legumes like beans, lentils, and chickpeas

• tofu

• Nuts (apart from coconut)

• seeds like sesame, chia, pumpkin, and sunflower seeds

• grains such quinoa, buckwheat, oats, barley, and wheat

Calcium

Milk, cheese, and yoghurt are calcium-rich foods for lacto-vegetarians.

Vegans should consume these calcium-rich foods:

• Tofu that has been prepared with calcium salt (see the label)

• calcium-fortified soy or substitute milk beverages (look for 120 mg calcium per 100 mL).

1. Almonds the tahini

• Asian leafy greens like book choy

Iron

Harem and non-hem iron are the two forms of iron found in food. Non-harem iron is not as well absorbed as hemp iron.

Harem iron is found in foods including meat, poultry, and shellfish. Only non-haem iron is present in plant meals and eggs.

The body can still get enough iron from plant-based diets, but to maximize absorption, they should be combined with a vitamin C-rich food. Suitable iron sources include:

• Legumes like chickpeas, beans, and lentils

• tense tofu

2. tempeh

• Sunflower seeds and pumpkin seeds (also known as pepitas)

• Nuts, particularly almonds and cashews

• Wholegrain bread, brown rice, amaranth, quinoa, and cereals made with whole grains like oats or muesli

• stale apricots

• green peas, kale, broccoli, and other cruciferous veggies

You may better absorb non-harem iron by eating fruits or vegetables that are all rich in vitamin C with each meal. Take a bite:

• eating berries, kiwis, melon, or having a rare, little glass of orange juice for breakfast.

• For lunch, choose a salad, homemade vegetable soup, or fresh fruit.

• At supper, vegetables like broccoli, capsicum, cabbage, cauliflower, snow peas, kale, pumpkin, spinach, or tomatoes

To replenish the iron lost in blood up until menopause, when menstruation ceases, persons who menstruate (also known as your period) require nearly twice as much iron as those who do not.

Even though they are better at absorbing non-harem iron, pregnant women need even more iron. Consult your doctor about obtaining a blood test if you're worried about your iron levels.

B12 vitamin

Blood formation is aided by vitamin B12, which also permits healthy nervous system operation. Animal products including milk, cheese, yoghurt, and eggs contain this vitamin. Some soy or alternative milk beverages and breakfast cereals also include it. Vegetarians need to include these items in their diet.

Vegans must take supplements in the form of dietary sources of vitamin B12 or injections to make up for the lack of vitamin B12 in their diets. Eating B12-fortified foods, such as certain morning cereals and some soy or alternative milk beverages, is an option. Verify if they are enriched with vitamin B12 by looking at the label.

There are no sources of vitamin B12 in spirulina, unfortified nutritional yeast, comfrey, tempeh, or mushrooms.

The omega 3 fats

Omega 3 is crucial for overall health and aids in illness prevention.

Long-chain omega-3 fats must come from your food since they are very rare in our bodies.

Fish, seafood, and seaweed all contain long chain omega 3 fatty acids. Short-chain omega-3 fats are also present in hemp, chia, and flax seeds and oils.

To ensure they get adequate long-chain omega-3 fats, vegans may take an algal-based omega-3 supplement.

Vegetarians who are pregnant or nursing, as well as small children, should take an omega-3 supplement.

Nutrition D

For strong bones and a healthy immune system, you need vitamin D.

The easiest way to get vitamin D is to expose your skin to sunlight for 15 minutes each day.

A source of vitamin D is eggs. Some fortified plant-based dairy products (like milk and margarine) also include vitamin D.

Is it okay for my kid to eat vegetarian food?

Children may follow a lacto-ovo vegetarian diet as long as they get a variety of plant foods.

Before placing kids on a vegan diet, particularly infants and toddlers, it's a good idea to see a doctor or dietician for guidance to make sure they're getting all the nutrients they need.

Inadequate nutrition brought on by a limited diet, if not well planned, may result in stunted development and vitamin deficiencies in children.

For the first two years, breast milk is healthiest for babies and toddlers. To ensure that young children getting started on a vegetarian or vegan diet receive adequate nutrients, seek expert counsel.

Do I need to see a dietitian?

If you wish to begin a vegetarian or vegan diet, it is essential to speak with a dietician. A nutritionist should be consulted if:

• You want to switch to a vegan diet.

• You want a kid or toddler to eat a vegan or vegetarian diet.

• You've previously had iron insufficiency.

• You are nursing, pregnant, or contemplating becoming pregnant.

Advice for vegans and vegetarians

• Consume 5 handfuls of veggies and 2 pieces of fruit each day.

• Consume a range of plant-based foods, such as wholegrain breads and cereals, legumes, nuts, seeds, and beans.

• Ensure that your milk alternatives are calcium-enriched.

• Check your iron levels.

• If you consume a vegan diet, take a vitamin B12 supplement as well.

Chapter 8

Summary

A vegetarian diet is beneficial to your health. Lowering a person's blood pressure, weight, cholesterol, and risk of cardiovascular disease development may all be beneficial. Additionally, it aids in the prevention of fatal chronic conditions like cancer and diabetes. It could also aid in extending lifetime. However, if the diet is not well organized, it may end up being detrimental to health. Therefore, further research should be done to demonstrate the advantages of a vegetarian diet. In my view, if someone is at risk of contracting a condition like diabetes, cardiovascular disease, kidney stones, hyperlipidemia, cataracts, or is experiencing depression, they should think about switching to a vegetarian diet as an alternative to adjuvant medication.

To ensure that vegetarian meals are nutritiously sufficient and healthy, they should be designed in line with the DRI or other authoritative nutritional recommendations. The nutrients that are likely to be deficient on unintended vegetarian diets are often different from those on unplanned omnivore diets. In certain instances, nutritional guidance and the right food choices may quickly and effectively correct these deficiencies. In others, it might be challenging to implement healthy eating habits due to ideological differences towards life, food, and nutrient requirements. By identifying high-risk individuals through nutritional status screening, identifying appropriate food sources of particular nutrients that may be lacking in the vegetarian's diet, suggesting dietary modifications that may be necessary to meet individual needs when intakes are insufficient, and tracking the vegetarian's progress, nutrition scientists and healthcare professionals can assist vegetarians who seek their advice.

The deliberate, voluntary decision to exclude one or more forms of animal products from the diet is known as vegetarianism. All types of vegetarian diets and vegetarians are together referred to as vegetarians. Ovo-lacto vegetarian diets, which allowed dairy products and eggs, and vegan diets, which forbid the use of any animal products, are two examples of different levels of vegetarianism. Regardless of the form of vegetarianism, someone who rigorously sticks to their vegetarian diet is referred to as a strict vegetarian.

The heterogeneity in diet composition, the use of "self-defined" vegetarians rather than a definition based on a dietary inventory, confounding by dietary and lifestyle characteristics that are associated with following a vegetarian diet, and lack of representativeness of the study population in the vast majority of published studies are methodological pitfalls in interpreting the literature on the health effects of vegetarian diets. It is quite challenging to come to reliable conclusions on the impact of vegetarian diets on health because of these methodological shortcomings.

Motives for Choosing a Vegetarian Diet

People choose for vegetarian diets for a variety of reasons. Health concerns are the primary driver of vegetarian diet adoption in western nations. Some people think that avoiding animal products is good for your health because it lowers your risk of contracting bacteria or other foodborne illnesses (like bovine spongiform encephalopathy), which are more likely to occur when animal products are prepared unhygienically or when you consume too much saturated fat, cholesterol, or sodium.

Others concentrate on the purported health advantages of plant-based diets, which not only include nutrients but also phytochemicals like fiber, flavonoids, and other substances that could have health advantages that are not yet fully understood. People who identify as "ethical vegetarians" often do so because to strong moral beliefs, such as their objection to the killing of animals for food or to what they see as the cruel treatment of farm animals. Others follow religions that support vegetarian eating habits, such as Seventh-Day Adventists, Buddhists, certain Hindus, and other religious sects, or subscribe to ideologies that promote vegetarianism among its adherents (such as transcendental meditators and anthroposophist's). Others are driven by environmental concerns, such as the belief that keeping animals for food uses resources that might be used to grow plant foods instead. And last, some people choose vegetarian diets just out of habit. In developing nations, vegetarian eating habits may arise from one or more of these causes, as well as from the fact that certain demographic groups cannot afford or get animal products.

The level of compliance with the selected vegetarian eating pattern relies on factors including motivation, habits, and environment. Until recently, the amount of avoiding animal foods and the divergence in other habits from omnivores could frequently be expected. As a result, vegans often hold beliefs that forbid not just the widespread use of dietary items derived from or used by animals (such as honey, casein, whey, rennet, and gelatin), but also the use of animal goods like leather, wool, or silk as well as the treatment of animals with kindness. The connections between nutrition and belief, however, are weaker now. Some vegans just concentrate on the eating style because they believe it has health benefits, but they may not adhere to all of the other standard vegan lifestyle and belief tenets. It is simpler to achieve nutritional sufficiency since they are more inclined to adopt meat substitutes, nutrient-fortified meals, and vitamin and mineral supplements.

A viable alternative to traditional dietary therapies for T2D is a vegetarian diet. Official position statements recommend that the transition to a vegetarian diet be managed by a skilled registered dietitian and a licensed physician. Vegetarian diets that are well designed are nutritiously sufficient, beneficial for controlling blood sugar levels and weight, and less likely to cause diabetic problems. They are long-term maintainable and may result in positive changes to both physical and mental health. In order to support the inclusion of vegetarian diets in dietary recommendations for the prevention and treatment of T2D, larger clinical studies are required to establish their efficacy.

Diabetes

Diets that are vegetarian encourage insulin sensitivity and glycemic management. This has been theorized to be caused by dietary elements that impact diabetes, such as consumption of fat, low calorie intake ratios, and high intakes of iron, magnesium, and vegetable protein. The vegetarian diet was shown to be related adversely with diabetes and impaired fasting glucose in menopausal women in a study of Taiwanese Buddhist postmenopausal vegetarians (OR for diabetes: 0.25, 95% CI: 0.15-0.42; OR for IFG: 0.73, 95% CI: 0.56-0.95). After controlling for a number of possible confounding variables, vegetarian diets were shown to have a robust protective effect against impaired fasting glucose and diabetes, but not in premenopausal women. The research revealed that owing to variations in vegetarian diet types, vegetarian diet durations, and study subject BMI, it was challenging to determine the impact of vegetarian diets on diabetes in pre- and postmenopausal women. Overall, it is challenging to come to consistent findings on how vegetarian diets affect postmenopausal women's risk for CVD and diabetes. On the basis of the nutritional makeup of vegetarian diets, there is a need for precise research that can pinpoint the beneficial benefits of vegetarian diets on several health concerns and can establish the link between estrogen levels and CVD risk. In the treatment of conditions including obesity, cancer, renal illness, RA, metabolic syndrome, diabetes, and cardiovascular disease, among others, vegetarian diets may be beneficial. Diets that are vegetarian are linked to lower rates of obesity, better weight reduction, a decreased risk of cardiovascular disease, and a lower overall mortality rate. Vegetarian diets may show potential as adjuvant therapy in the treatment of illness, given the growing body of research demonstrating the health advantages of plant-based diets. Vegetarian diets are being studied more and more in terms of how they affect the gut microbiota, which in turn affects disease states via regulating inflammation.

Understanding the processes that connect nutrition and health and determining whether short-term diet treatment may have long-term positive effects on health need further investigation.

Vegan and vegetarian diets

Vegan diets are those that exclude any food that comes from animals, whereas vegetarian diets vary in their content. Due in part to their usually superior nutritional quality, vegetarian diets are often believed to improve health. Vegetarian diets tend to be higher in fiber and lower in protein than omnivore diets, which creates a balance that promotes saccharolytic fermentation as opposed to proteolytic fermentation. Conducted a systematic review of the associations between vegetarian or vegan diets and the composition of the microbiota. They found no associations between omnivores and vegetarian or vegan diet consumers' microbiomes, and they came to the conclusion that the high inter-individual variability precluded the description of a typical vegetarian or vegan microbiome profile. In one such research, indicate in their cross-sectional analysis that the number of Bactericides in the microbiomes of vegetarians, vegans, and omnivores may vary; nevertheless, generalizations about the makeup of the gut microbiota cannot be drawn merely based on dietary pattern. Barrett et al. recently compared women who ate an omnivore or vegetarian diet in the first trimester of pregnancy. They discovered that vegetarians had somewhat lower beta diversity but not alpha diversity. They also discovered that they had lower abundances of Collinsella and Hold mania but greater abundances of Roseboro and Lachnospiraceae. In conclusion, eating a vegetarian diet does not appear to produce a distinctive microbiome profile, which may partly be attributable to the dietary variety of vegetarian diets. As a result, the microbiome profile may not be the only mechanism by which this dietary pattern has health benefits. However, whether vegan, vegetarian, or omnivore, food type also affects how the microbiome functions metabolically. Vegans and vegetarians have larger concentrations of microbial genes and proteins that are involved in processes like the breakdown of polysaccharides and proteins and the creation of vitamins.